Copyright © James W. Abbott

All rights reserved.

First Kindle Edition: 9th September 2013

ISBN-13: 978-149271265-7
ISBN-10: 149271265-5

Table of Contents

Talking to Your Dentist

Dental Economics

Treatment Devices

Cast Gold Crowns

Porcelain Fused to Metal

Porcelain Fused to Gold-Infiltrated High-Noble Alloy

Porcelain Fused to Zirconia

Monolithic Zirconia

Monolithic Lithium-Disilicate

Feldspathic Layered Porcelain "Veneers"

Porcelain Fused to Lithium-Disilicate

Porcelain Fused to Fully-Sintered Alumina

Porcelain Fused to Glass-Infiltrated Alumina

Asking for What You Want

Summary

Trademark References

Talking to Your Dentist

Chances are your dentist is a busy guy. Dental practice today, is very competitive. Over time, practice has become more and more business oriented. So if you want to talk to your dentist about any treatment that you want or that he recommends, you had better do your homework. His practice appoints his time by the quarter hour and the topic of treatment options fills textbooks. Moreover, each dentist has his "routine" and may or may not be comfortable offering some services.

That said, you can get what you want if you just know how to ask for it.

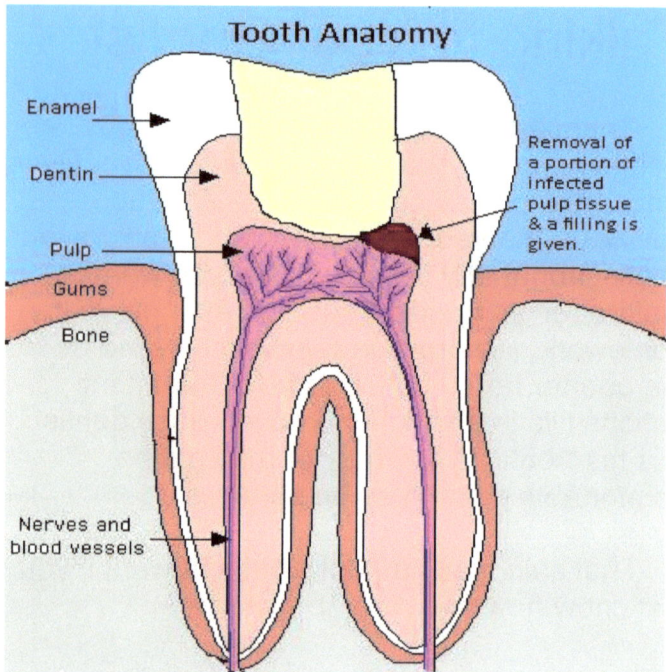

Pulpotomy image credit:
http://www.intelligentdental.com

 When someone goes to a dentist they usually go for a biannual cleaning – if nothing is identified as needing treatment, then the patient may not be seeing the dentist again for another 6 months. Otherwise, a person goes to the dentist because there is pain somewhere in their mouth. If there is pain, and dental treatment is required to alleviate it, then the patient may become involved in the first of three steps that are the dental treatment steps:

STEP 1. Temporary alleviation of pain (such as, injecting a local anesthetic, removing the pulp core of a tooth, temporarily filling the resulting gap, and prescribing an antibiotic).

STEP 2. Permanent correction of the defect that caused pain (such as, doing a root canal and permanently filling the gap).

STEP 3. Restoration of function and cosmetic defects (such as, drilling down the tooth to form a tapered stump that can be covered with a cemented permanent crown).

Mostly, dentistry is a labor-intensive hand-crafts field of work. There are no shortcuts. But there are time/motion efficiencies and you will probably notice that when you are in your dentist's chair, everything keeps moving right along. This is because "chairtime," as it is called, is not cheap.

So one thing to keep in mind is, when you are in the chair talking about your treatment, always communicate as clearly and concisely as you can. Do your homework before you are at your Step 3 appointment. If dental crown options have not already been discussed and agreed upon, telephone your dentist and talk to him about the restorative devices and options that you want. Make sure that you document this conversation in your own records and when he agrees to your requested device options, you can and should request that the dentist enter this information in your "chart." Most patients know nothing about restorative devices, options, and costs. They coast through their Step 3 appointment with little or no dialog about dental crown options.

After the Step 3 appointment, this conversation is too late – the prescription describing what the dentist wants will already have been written and the case materials will have been sent to one of the dentist's labs. By the time you arrive for your Step 3 appointment, you and your dentist should already have had a discussion and reached agreement about your treatment device design, materials, and point of origin (if you don't want your device made in China or some other third world country, you will have to make that known).

The Food and Drug Administration and the American Dental Association are currently investigating reports of lead in imported dental work. It is estimated that 7 million crowns a year are made offshore. According to recent reports, some dental patients are becoming ill with 160 to 210 parts per million lead content in their crown and bridge materials (both metal and porcelain materials). By comparison, children's toys having 90 parts per million have been recalled for being unsafe. Patients should always ask their dentist where their crowns are made and what the material contents are (metal, ceramic, and porcelain). However, many dentists have no way of knowing for sure what the material contents are. Domestic labs often send work off shore and there is no law that requires them to disclose to the patient where the work was made. Some of these labs are even printing fake materials labels that are affixed to packaging of the delivered devices.

Dental Economics

In the U.S. the "usual and customary" fee for one crown is about $1,000. But fees may be as low as $500 and as high as $5,000. High-end dentists strive for a superior reputation and skill set. Few dentists achieve these aspirations because dental practice requires diverse skills, including mechanical, cosmetic, scientific, and management skills.

Better dentists are often perfectionists who enjoy close relations with lab technicians (the people who fabricate their treatment devices). These traits are the best indicators of a dentist with high standards.

A few artistically inclined dentists specialize in aesthetic (cosmetic) dentistry – almost all dentists advertise this skill, but few actually deliver it. Some mechanically inclined dentists specialize in instrument oriented dentistry (T.M.J., occlusion, or gnathology), but again, professing to specialize is not a guarantee that the dentist is delivering a high standard service. Some dentists have fellowship and academic credentials. While credentials, teaching affiliations, and speaking engagements, do indicate peer status and accomplishments, these are no assurance patients are getting a higher standard-of-care.

   Depending on how much extra time the dentist spends working with patients, instruments, measurements, and stone models, his fee could be understandably higher. Depending on where the dentist practices, the fee could be higher or lower simply because of overhead costs and staff compensation needs. Rule of thumb, the fancier and bigger the practice layout, the more you will pay – and sometimes the layout really does indicate high restorative treatment standards. On the other hand, a modest office that is clean and well-organized often means you may get more value in terms of your treatment. Generally, dentists who do not scrimp on the lab bill tend to produce better treatment outcomes.

In most cases your dentist has to order and buy your restoration from a third party, a dental lab, where the restoration (device) must be fabricated according your dentist's prescription. The device which he will provide for you will cost your dentist about $150. A high-end lab may charge upwards of $300 to make a crown. If you opt for an upgrade, any lab-to-dentist amount in excess of $150 may be added to your dentist-to-patient fee. So if you and your dentist agree to send your case to a high-end lab with an exceptional porcelain artist (ceramist) doing **"layered porcelain,"** you may have to pay $150 more to cover the added cost of a high aesthetic crown. All labs in the U.S. collect their fees from the dentists they work for, so unless you ask for a copy of the lab bill, you will never see it.

Primarily, dentistry in the U.S. is a "fee for service" occupation. That is, people who have "dental insurance plans" that actually pay the dentist for a portion of his fee are uncommon. Mostly, these plans are provided in whole or in part by employers. When plan rules are followed this insurance pays for cleanings twice yearly and a percentage of treatment costs. Today the percent paid for treatments is around 50%.

Then there are "dental discount plans" that are really not insurance at all. These discount plans appear to pay as much as 50% of the costs, but in reality the plans are part of a marketing scheme that requires the dentist to discount his services by as much as 50%. Why would a dentist discount his fees that much? He does this in exchange for large numbers of patients that are referred to his practice by mass marketing techniques such as internet advertising and third-party websites. Dentists participating in these plans agree in advance, to discount any patient who shows up with a valid dental (discount) card. The patient pays a nominal monthly fee to the marketing company to keep the card active, which fee is designed to cover the company's marketing expenses plus profit.

Obviously, dentists who discount their fees are going to have to shave off expenses somewhere just to stay in business. In practice, attempts to hold down costs almost always result in treatment device flaws.

Take for example, the crown with a "catch." This is a common flaw in substandard dental work. You won't notice a catch until you have lived with it a while. A catch collects food and is difficult to impossible to clean. Resulting in bad breath, decay, and even systemic diseases, such as diabetes and heart disease, a catch is the result of careless clinical work and cheap lab work.

Remember, dentistry is a labor-intensive field of work. Patients in many discount practices complain about a lot of different things. But, consistently, most everything they complain about is related directly or indirectly to a practice's need to reduce the time and resources normally required for patient care. Ironically, even in the better practices, sometimes treatments are rushed, often leading to disappointed patients.

This leads us to the recommended patient motto, *"NEVER RUSH THE DENTIST OR THE*

LAB." If you need a dental restoration in time for a special event or a trip, always allow at least two months to completion. It may take you two months just to get in for the first appointment, so you probably should call your dentist's office four months ahead of the scheduled event. That way, if there are problems along the way, you are not put into the position of asking for a "rush job." Some practices are always rushing treatments, and patients in these practices are not getting the best care. As a staff member in one of these practices put it, "We never have time to do it right – but we always make time to do it over."

Treatment Devices

Dental restorative devices can be grouped into two classes; fixed (such as a cemented crown or bridge); and removable (such as a patient-removable partial or complete denture). This book is concerned only with fixed crowns, bridges (crowns connected to pontics that replace missing teeth), veneer-facings (a thin aesthetic covering bonded to the facial surface of a front tooth), and inlays (cemented fillings). Implants are restored with fixed and removable devices, but implants will be the topic of a future ebook. Fixed treatment devices are primarily fabricated utilizing one or more of the following materials; feldspathic porcelain; alumina (with or without infiltration glass); lithium disilicate; zirconia; gold; platinum; palladium; silver; chrome cobalt; nickel; trace metals; and composite resin. Some materials cost more than others and this may have a small impact the cost of treatment.

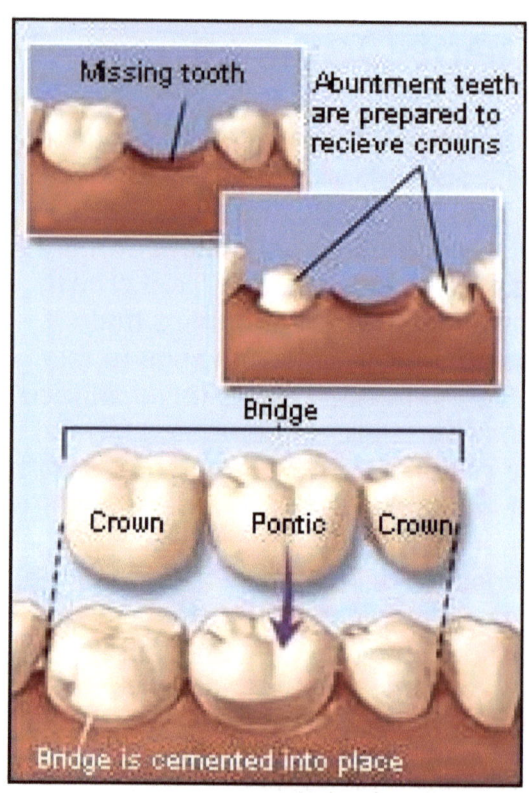

Dental Bridge image credit:
http://www.webmd.com

Dental restorative materials can be grouped into two classes; monolithic (such as all-zirconia ceramic crowns or all-gold alloy crowns); and veneered (such as porcelain fused to alloy crowns or porcelain fused to zirconia crowns).

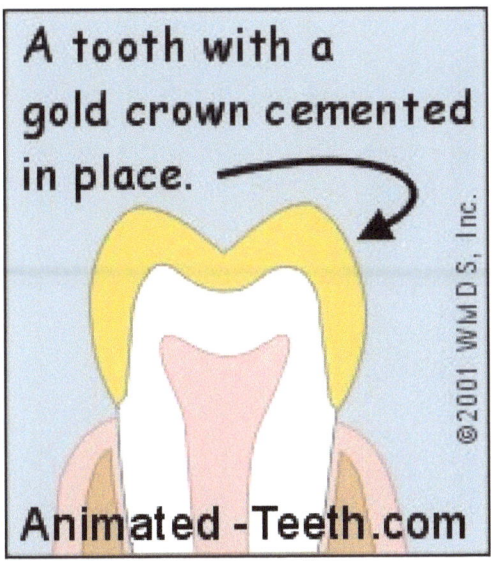

Dental Crown image credit:
http://www.animated-teeth.com

In recent years, the field of dentistry has increasingly become cluttered with devices and materials having short track records and uncertain sponsorship and countries of origin. Many of these products are heavily promoted to dentists by companies primarily focused on reducing costs with little regard for the patient's standard-of-care. This book has been written to help patients avoid some of the risks associated with these products.

Cast Gold Crowns

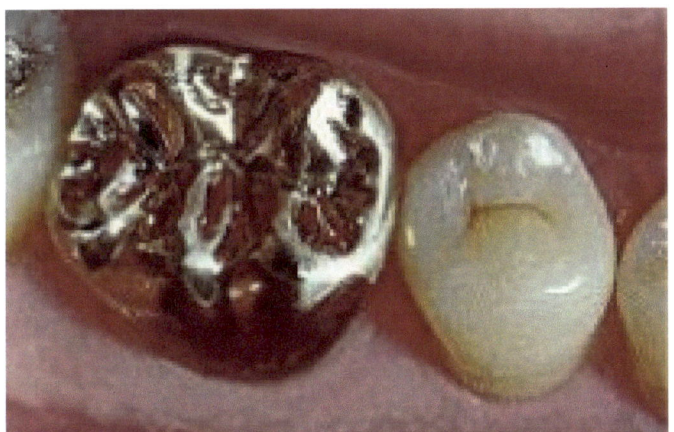

Cast Gold Crown

    Traditionally, crowns and bridges in the back of the mouth (posterior) were made of **cast gold alloy**. The yellow color metal has been used for dental work since Etruscan times. Gold is well respected by dentists who still like this restoration for its durability (this crown can not fracture) and ductility and they often prescribe it in their own mouths. It is said to be more "gentle to periodontal support mechanisms," that is, gentler to the teeth, gum, and bone support areas in the mouth.

The only drawback for gold is most people do not like it to show. So, molar teeth are a safe choice for gold crowns. If you need a bridge and want it in gold, the second bicuspid can be used as a crown abutment and most people will not notice it when you smile. The cost of cast gold is usually comparable to other tooth-colored materials. Inlays are often made of cast gold. Cast gold crown survival rates are more than 10 years.

Porcelain Fused to Metal

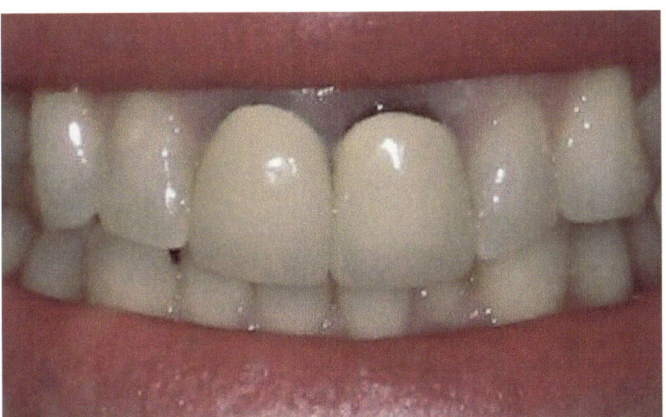

Two Porcelain Fused to Metal Crowns image credit: http://www.darrengardner-dds.com

    The next most traditional restorative device is the **porcelain fused to metal (PFM) crown**. The "metal" is one of hundreds of dental alloys ranging from high-gold to silver-palladium to nonprecious (predominantly base metal) alloys. The metal serves as a support structure for the crown or bridge. The porcelain serves as an aesthetic veneer that causes the restoration to look like natural teeth.

Although this device can have very aesthetic properties, it has two faults; (1) the metal core is not at all translucent (light passes through healthy natural teeth and this property gives teeth their enigmatic beauty), so a PFM crown may not look good in all lighting conditions; and (2) the gumline can show a black oxide that becomes more and more noticeable over the years as gums and bone pull away from the oxidized crown margin.

The metal core is strong. Bond strength to veneer porcelain is good. Dental cement adhesion is excellent. Porcelain fused to metal crown survival rates are more than 10 years.

Porcelain Fused to Gold-Infiltrated High-Noble Alloy

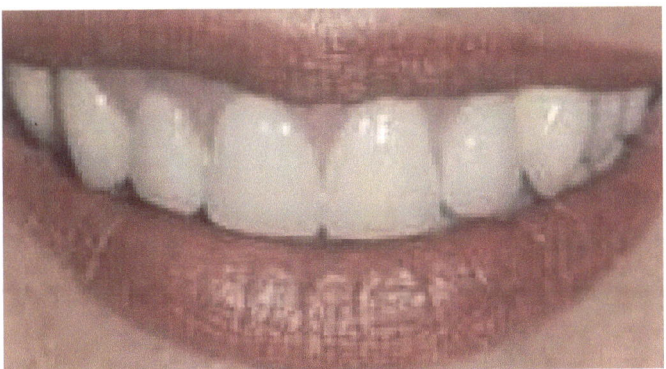

Six (Anterior) *Captek* Crowns

Porcelain fused to a bioactive support structure has become very popular in recent years. The material that is most respected, with a 20-year track record, is **porcelain fused to gold-infiltrated high-noble alloy (called *Captek*[1])**. Of all the dental materials and technologies, this one has the capacity of improving surrounding gum tissue health. If you have a "gummy smile," this crown can have real aesthetic advantages. Moreover, this crown has important health advantages for people who suffer from gum tissue and bone support issues (such as periodontal disease) because gum problems can lead to serious systemic problems like heart disease.

This crown has excellent fit on prepared tooth stumps. Fit is important because this keeps decay from tunneling in under your crown.

Many cosmetic dentists say, *Captek* crowns have excellent aesthetics – although the metal core is not translucent, the yellow gold color of the core reflects light much like the core of a natural tooth, and this imparts a warm glow that is entirely believable.

The metal core is strong because it combines a tough gold-platinum-palladium-silver alloy scaffold with resilient yellow gold infiltration. A yellow gold bonder produces superior bond strength to veneer porcelain.

Dental cement adhesion is excellent. *Captek* crown survival rates are more than 10 years.

Porcelain Fused to Zirconia

Since the introduction of advanced ceramic support structures, porcelain fused to ceramic has been gaining market share over PFM crowns. One of these new support structures is zirconia. At one time the fastest growing dental crown, the **porcelain fused to zirconia crown (some called *Lava*[2])** has more recently lost market share because of fractures and crumbling of zirconia's veneer porcelain. Zirconia, being one of the hardest known ceramic materials, is stronger than any other dental ceramic. But, in comparing porcelain veneer bond strength to other dental materials, zirconia's bond is significantly lower. So, while the zirconia support structures are strong, the porcelain veneer has been found to chip and crumble within 3 to 5 years of placement in significant numbers of cases.

Because zirconia needs to be milled, fit of porcelain fused to zirconia crowns is not as good as some other crown modalities. Fit is important because this keeps decay from tunneling in under your crown.

For a metal-free crown, these restorations are not translucent so they don't always look very natural in the front of the mouth. Porcelain fused to zirconia crown survival rates are generally 3 to 5 years.

Monolithic Zirconia

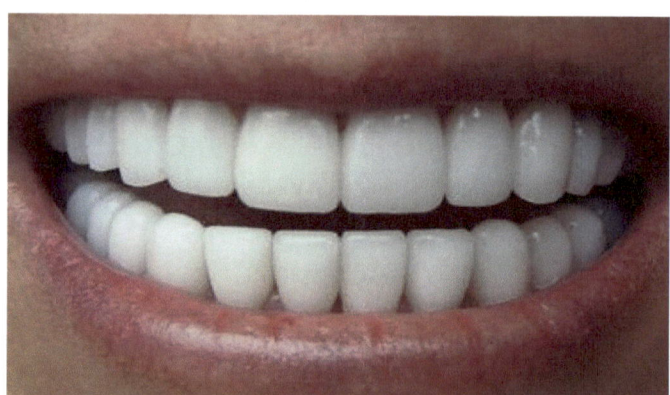

Monolithic Zirconia Crowns

Currently, a more popular zirconia crown modality is the **zirconia monolithic crown (some called *BruxZir³*)**. This crown is made entirely of zirconia (no veneer porcelain). The monolithic zirconia crown is not very esthetic but it is strong and costs the dentist less than most any other crown. Stains are needed to make shades look a little more like natural teeth. Zirconia materials are not translucent and, even the new "translucent" generations of these materials are really not very translucent at all.

Not suitable for use in the front of the mouth (anterior), this crown is a good choice in the back of the mouth (posterior) because it is way stronger than any other dental ceramic material.

Since zirconia needs to be milled, fit of monolithic zirconia crowns is not as good as cast gold crowns. As a relatively new product, zirconia monolithic crown survival rates are estimated at more than 10 years.

Monolithic Lithium-Disilicate

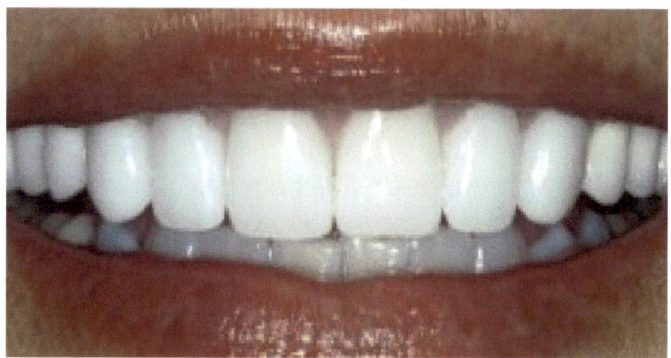

Monolithic *E.max Press* Crowns

    The fastest growing crown product today is the **lithium-disilicate monolithic crown (called *e.max Press*[4] or *e.max CAD*[4])**. Made entirely of lithium disilicate material (no veneer porcelain), this crown is also not very esthetic and costs the dentist less to have made by labs. But superficial (surface) stains can be applied and the incisal (edge of a front tooth) can be cut back and layered with veneer porcelain to make shades look a little more natural.

Each shade is available in different translucencies. Standard shades can be too gray and light shades tend to have a bright unnatural, glassy look. If you like unnatural gleaming white smiles, monolithic *e.max* may be your best option. (The author's next book will talk about dental shades and what to avoid in "bleaching" your teeth and choosing a "shade.")

Lithium-disilicate monolithic crowns are made by "pressing" heated material into a mould or by "milling" blocks of solid material in a dental milling machine – fit of pressed *e.max* crowns is better than fit of the milled *e.max* crowns. These crowns are not as strong as zirconia monolithic crowns, but they are stronger than porcelain fused crowns. *E.max* has excellent bond strength to the cement used to hold it in place. One reason *e.max* is prescribed by so many dentists – it is often produced at a lower cost by high-volume production labs. Inlays (small cemented fillings) can be made of lithium-disilicate, which is a good material for this purpose. Veneer-facings (thin cosmetic coverings for the facial surfaces of front teeth) are also made of lithium-disilicate, although better results can be achieved with feldspathic porcelain veneer-facings. As a new material, lithium-disilicate monolithic crown survival rates are estimated at about 10 years.

Feldspathic Layered Porcelain "Veneers"

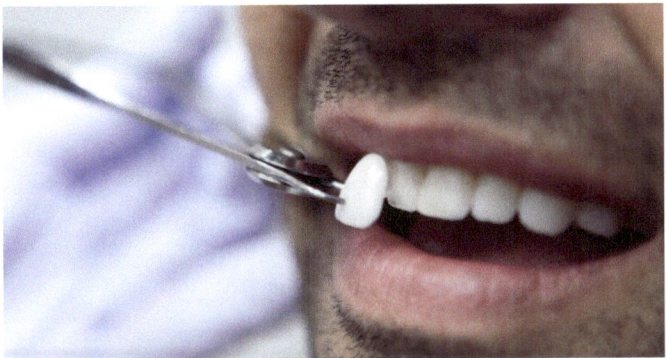

Layered Porcelain Veneer-Facing image credit:
http://www.durathinveneers.com

Though the material is not new, feldspathic porcelain was found to be bondable to tooth enamel in the 1980's. Since then, people looking to improve their smile have been paying out of pocket (not reimbursed by any dental plan) for **feldspathic layered porcelain veneer-facings (some are called Lumineers[5])**. "Veneers" as they are often called, are high-end to low-end treatments.

Sometimes they are delivered as a low-cost alternative to crowns. But some dentists, more correctly, see them as challenging cosmetic treatments, reserved for the patient who can afford the very best cosmetic treatment on front teeth that are otherwise healthy.

Like all restorative devices, veneers have two cost variables; (1) the dentist's reputation and skill set; (2) the fabricating lab's reputation and skill set. When well done, veneers are excellent alternatives to dental crowns, requiring less cutting down of the natural tooth and appearing entirely natural. However, well done veneers can be very expensive because they require more knowledge and skill on the part of the dentist and his lab. When poorly done, veneers can look artificial.

Because veneers are bonded to only the front half of the tooth, they can stick out in functional areas and cause excessive wear against opposing teeth and unpredictable breakage of the veneer and/or the prepared tooth. Well done feldspathic porcelain veneer-facing survival rates are more than 10 years.

Porcelain Fused to Lithium-Disilicate

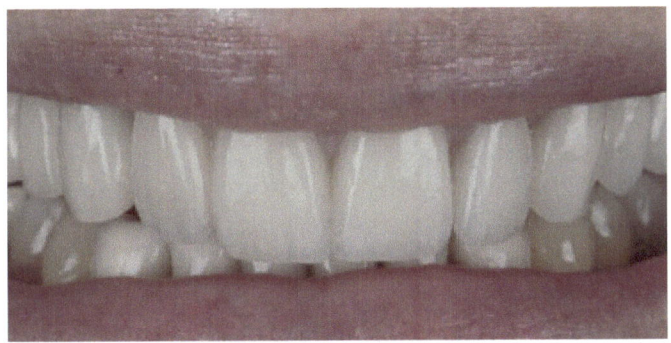

Layered Porcelain *E.max Ceram* Crowns image credit: http://lakeforestdentalarts.com

    The **porcelain fused to lithium-disilicate crown (called *e.max Empress* and *e.max Ceram*[4])** is the porcelain (glass-ceramic) veneered version of *e.max*. Less common because it is a higher cost upgrade, dentists prescribing "*e.max*" are more commonly referring to the low-cost monolithic version of the product. This porcelain veneered *e.max* crown is not as strong as monolithic *e.max*. But porcelain veneer bond strength is excellent and bond strength to cement (used to hold it in place) is higher than other porcelain fused crowns.

Lithium-disilicate material is formed into support structures (for porcelain fused crowns) by "pressing" heated material into a mould (*e.max Empress*) or by "milling" blocks of solid material in a dental milling machine (*e.max Ceram*) – fit of the pressed *e.max* support structures is better than fit of the milled *e.max* support structures. Porcelain fused to lithium disilicate crowns are very aesthetic – one of few crowns that is suitable for use in the anterior. As a new material, the porcelain fused to lithium-disilicate crown survival rates are estimated at about 10 years.

Porcelain Fused to Fully-Sintered Alumina

The **porcelain fused to fully-sintered alumina crown (called *ProCera*[6])** was introduced in the late 1990's. Because this alumina needs to be milled, fit of porcelain fused to fully-sintered alumina crowns is not as good as some other crown modalities. But porcelain fused to sintered alumina crowns are very aesthetic – suitable for use in the anterior. Crowns have consistent translucency.

The material is strong, but without any infiltration-glass, porcelain veneer bond strength is significantly lower and bond strength to dental cement not so good. Alumina is the only permanent restorative material that is radiolucent – that is, when the dentist takes an x-ray of your teeth, alumina is the only material that will let him see if the natural tooth underneath is healthy and decay free. Fully sintered alumina crown survival rates are more than 7 years.

Porcelain Fused to Glass-Infiltrated Alumina

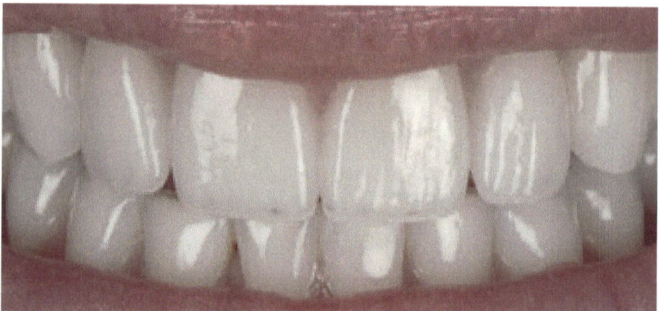

Six (Anterior) Layered Porcelain *Wol-Ceram* Crowns

    Porcelain fused to ceramic support structures have become very popular in recent years. The material that is most respected, with a 20-year track record, is **porcelain fused to glass-infiltrated alumina (called *Wol-Ceram*[7] and *In-Ceram*[8])**. Of all the dental materials and technologies, this one has the closest and most consistently accurate fit on prepared tooth stumps. Fit is important because this keeps decay from tunneling in under your crown. It has consistently excellent translucency.

Many leading cosmetic dentists say porcelain fused to glass-infiltrated alumina crowns set the standard for aesthetics in dentistry – one of few crowns that is suitable for use in the anterior.

The material is strong and, because it has infiltration-glass, bond strength to veneer porcelain and dental cement is excellent. Alumina is the only permanent restorative material that is radiolucent – that is, when the dentist takes an x-ray of your teeth, alumina is the only material that will let him see if the natural tooth underneath is healthy and decay free. Glass-infiltrated alumina crown survival rates are more than 10 years.

Asking for What You Want

Dental crown and bridge devices are either best in the anterior (front) or best in the posterior (back) of the mouth. Some low-cost devices, such as monolithic *e.max* and monolithic zirconia, are more or less tooth-colored and very strong – but they lack the look of natural teeth and so should only be placed in the back of the mouth. Cast gold is virtually indestructible and it is kinder to the teeth, gum, and bone support areas – but cast gold crowns are also not very aesthetic so they should also be placed in the back.

Comparing all the other choices, the most aesthetic crowns are (1) the porcelain fused to glass-infiltrated alumina crown (*Wol-Ceram* or *In-Ceram*), (2) the porcelain fused to gold-infiltrated high-noble alloy crown (*Captek*), and (3) the porcelain fused to lithium-disilicate crown (*e.max Empress* and *e.max Ceram* – but one has to be careful when asking for *"e.max,"* not to inadvertently end up with any of the other *e.max* monolithic products that are not very aesthetic at all). To make cosmetic improvements on healthy teeth (teeth that are not broken or otherwise defective), layered porcelain veneers are a good restorative solution.

Leading cosmetic dentists agree, monolithic lithium disilicate (*e.max Press* and *e.max CAD*) and monolithic zirconia (*BruxZir* and other brands) may be good options for posterior teeth – but monolithic crowns are not usually the best choice in the anterior region because of aesthetic concerns; Dr. Ed McLaren, *"…a monolithic restoration that is surface stained… still lacks that three-dimensional effect that the layered restoration offers…;"* Dr. Robert Margeas, *"I prefer only layered restorations in the anterior region…;"* Dr. Newton Fahl, *"Feldspathic [layered] veneers are, however, my primary choice in most cases because I can achieve better and consistent aesthetics with minimum tooth reduction."** Bottom line –

layered porcelain is still the best option for anterior crowns.

If a top-notch ceramist is engaged to build **"layered porcelain,"** then for sure you will have the very best crown that is available in the dental marketplace today. But this may cost your dentist upwards of $300 (this is at least $150 more than most dentists pay). Low-cost monolithic crowns and crowns made in China are sold for as little as $50, so some dentists are accustomed to paying very little for their crowns.

The best approach to getting what you want from your dentist is to talk with him on the telephone before you need treatments. Simply ask if he can "deliver" the device that you want. Ask for only one or two device options. Do not attempt to show off your knowledge of treatment devices – let him lead you a little. Many dentists do not like treating patients with too much dental knowledge – often such patients fit a profile that is known in the field as "psychotic." Be humble. After all, he is the professional.

Keep the following list in front of you as your dentist talks about good and bad experiences he has had with any of these restorations:

☑ "Full Gold"
(Cast Gold Crowns)
BEST POSTERIOR T.M.J. CROWN

☐ "PFM"
(Porcelain Fused to Metal)

☑ "*Captek*"
(Porcelain Fused to Gold-Infiltrated High-Noble Alloy)
BEST GUM-HEALTH CROWN

☐ "Zirconia"
(Porcelain Fused to Zirconia)

☑ "*BruxZir*" – "Full Zirconia"
(Monolithic Zirconia)
BEST POSTERIOR COSMETIC CROWN

☐ "*e.max*" – "*e.max Press* or *e.max CAD*"

(Monolithic Lithium Disilicate)

☐ *"Lumineers"* – "Porcelain Veneers"
(Feldspathic Layered Porcelain "Veneers")

☑ *"e.max"* – "*e.max Empress* and *e.max Ceram"* – not *e.max Press* or *e.max CAD*
(Porcelain Fused to Lithium Disilicate*)*
GOOD ANTEROR COSMETIC CROWN

☐ *"ProCera"*
(Porcelain Fused to Fully-Sintered Alumina)

☑ *"Wol-Ceram"* – *"In-Ceram"*
(Porcelain Fused to
Glass-Infiltrated Alumina)
BEST ANTEROR COSMETIC CROWN

Listed are "common names" often used by dentists to refer to products they work with. Be prepared to ask for what you want again. If you feel stonewalled politely discontinue the conversation. Do not try to change your dentist's opinion. Do not seek leads for second opinions from your dentist (many dentists refer patients to collogues who they subsequently prompt to provide you with the like-minded information). Call other dentists (who are not working in the same office) to find out who delivers the treatment you want.

When you ask for a particular restorative device, do not be surprised if the dentist seems amazed. He does not see many patients who are concerned much about their own dental care – have you looked at other peoples smiles lately? Ad-hoc, he may not know if his labs make the product you are asking for or, he many not know how much he will have to pay for it. Let him know, "While I do not have unlimited resources, if we can agree on a small cost difference in lab work, I can pay the difference." If you live in a small town, be prepared to offer phone numbers of labs in the U.S. that you have talked to and that claim to make the product you want. Most dentists mail-order restorative devices from labs, so mailing should not be a problem.

Sadly, some dentists are too proud to work with patients seeking device options. You may have good reasons to trust your dentist implicitly. Just understand that as a dental patient, you will be paying, directly or indirectly, for restorative devices that are a significant part your dental treatments. Better quality devices will keep you healthier, improve your appearance, and be easier to keep clean.

If your dentist blocks your attempts to communicate, you do have options. When you are in this situation, you can find dentists who deliver the restorative devices you are looking for by asking dental companies (that make the device materials) for names of labs they sell to in your area (see Trademark References). Labs can refer you to the dentists they work with. It's like deciding that you want to buy a Ford and finding the Ford dealer in your area. Choose restorative devices wisely.

You have options. Historically, some patients have experienced less than satisfactory dental care by not knowing what to ask for and what to look for. Today, people are better informed consumers. Internet access has empowered people to investigate high ticket products and services like automobiles, appliances and dental treatments. For additional information, contact the author by email – jmsabbott@live.com. To comment on Amazon Kindle Book Forum, connect to link – https://www.google.com/url?sa=t&rct=j&q=&esrc=s&source=web&cd=2&cad=rja&ved=0CDgQFjAB&url=http%3A%2F%2Fwww.amazon.com%2Fforum%2Fkindle%2520book%3F_encoding%3DUTF8%26cdForum%3DFx3RFWX8IMGF85E&ei=ufj7UY3QMJCA9QS0oYCwDQ&usg=AFQjCNE6u-D6_Ddk5GEkRCLyEPE36cO94A&sig2=L-0jVGL0Am6fa0mUb0RpVA. This book has provided a basis for understanding dental restorative devices and related costs. With this information you can save on dental expenses, spend a little more to get the very best treatment outcomes, and identify high value options.

*Where and When Is It Appropriate to Place Monolithic vs. Layered Restorations, *Inside Dentistry*, August 2012, Vol. 8, Issue 8, E. McLaren, R. Margeas, and N. Fahl.

Summary

First and foremost, you need to see a dentist twice a year for a hygiene appointment and checkup. The dentist can advise you as to your homecare practices and dental health. About half of the U.S. population ignores the six-month rule. Not seeing a dentist twice a year can cost you more because problems that are caught early can often be fixed with simple chairside fillings that are comparatively much less expensive than crowns. In the 2012 Senate Report, *Dental Crisis in America*, the Institute of Medicine acknowledged that one fourth of adults in the U.S., age 65 and older, have lost all of their teeth. To avoid tooth loss over time, have six-month checkups. Choose your dentist and the treatment devices he delivers wisely:

Tip 1: Better dentists are often perfectionists who enjoy close relations with lab technicians (the people who fabricate their treatment devices).

Tip 2: A modest office that is clean and well-organized often means you may get more value in terms of your treatment.

Tip 3: Generally, dentists who do not scrimp on the lab bill tend to produce better treatment outcomes.

Tip 4: A few artistically inclined dentists specialize in aesthetic (cosmetic) dentistry – almost all dentists advertise a cosmetic service, but few actually deliver it.

Tip 5: Some mechanically inclined dentists specialize in instrument oriented dentistry (T.M.J., occlusion, or gnathology), but again, professing to specialize is not a guarantee that the dentist is delivering a functionally superior treatment result.

Tip 6: Some dentists have fellowship and academic credentials. While credentials, teaching affiliations, and speaking engagements, do indicate peer status and accomplishments, these are no assurance patients are getting a higher standard-of-care.

Tip 7: Depending on how much extra time the dentist spends working with patients, instruments, measurements, and stone models, his fee could be understandably higher.

Tip 8: In the posterior (back of the mouth), cast gold crowns are the most durable and healthy restorative option, while monolithic zirconia crowns are the most durable and aesthetic option.

Tip 9: In the anterior (front of the mouth), the best looking restorative devices have layered porcelain. Of these, the best options are (1) the porcelain fused to glass-infiltrated alumina crown (*Wol-Ceram* or *In-Ceram*), (2) the porcelain fused to gold-infiltrated high-noble alloy crown (*Captek*), and (3) the porcelain fused to lithium-disilicate crown (*e.max Empress* and *e.max Ceram* – but one has to be careful here, not to inadvertently end up with any of the other *e.max* monolithic products that are not very aesthetic at all). To make cosmetic improvements on healthy front teeth (teeth that are not broken or otherwise defective), layered porcelain veneers are a good restorative solution for closing gaps, correcting tooth shape and position, and improving tooth shades.

Tip 10: If your dentist blocks attempts to communicate, you can find dentists who deliver the restorative devices you are looking for by asking dental companies that make device materials (see Trademark References) for names of labs they sell to in your area. Labs can refer you to the dentists they work with.

Tip 11: Never rush the dentist or the lab – it is always better to give them extra time to deliver the treatment. The more time they allot to your case, the more likely you will be happy with the results.

Trademark References

1 *Captek*
   Argen Corporation
   5855 Oberlin Drive
   San Diego, CA 92121
   Phone: 800-255-5524

2 *Lava*
   3M ESPE
   3M Center
   St. Paul, MN 55144
   Phone: 888-364-3577

3 *BruxZir*
   Glidewell Labs
   4141 MacArther Boulevard
   Newport Beach, CA 92660
   Phone: 800-854-7256

4 *E.max*
   Invoclar Vivadent
   175 Pineview Drive West
   Amherst, NY 14228
   Phone: 716-691-1370

5 *Lumineers*
   DenMat
   1017 West Central Avenue
   Lompoc, CA 93436
   Phone: 805-922-8491

6 *ProCera*
   Nobel Biocare
   800 Corporate Drive
   Mahwah, NJ 07430
   Phone: 201-828-9250

7 *Wol-Ceram*
   Bio-CAM
   13833 Wellington Trace
   Suite E4-426
   West Palm Beach, FL 33414
   Phone: 561-333-6651

8 *In-Ceram*
   Vident
   3150 East Birch Street
   Brea, CA 92821
   Phone: 800-828-3839

Dental Crown Options:
How to Get What You Want from Your Dentist

James W. Abbott

ISBN-13: 978-149271265-7
ISBN-10: 149271265-5

www.ingramcontent.com/pod-product-compliance
Lightning Source LLC
Chambersburg PA
CBHW040858180526
45159CB00001B/459